Autism Uncovered:

A Look at the New Faces of Neurodiversity

By

Byron D. Johnson

Copyright © Byron D. Johnson 2022.

Table of content

Introduction

A thorough examination of the autistic experience spectrum and the phenomenon of masked autism will provide people with the knowledge they need to discover their actual selves securely and help society's limited grasp of neurodiversity.

"A fantastic piece of work that will lead the push for neurodiversity."

Numerous "masked" Autistic people pass for neurotypical for every autistic person you see who is visible. To conform to cultural norms, masking is a typical coping strategy used by autistic persons.

In doing so, they adopt a phony identity at the risk of their mental health. To avoid being perceived as needy or "strange," they may repress harmless stims and mask communication. Difficulties by being modest and mild-mannered or putting themselves in situations that make them highly anxious.

In Uncovering Autism, Byron D. Johnson combines history, social science research, medical advice, and individual profiles to create a story of neurodivergence that has so far been dominated by those on the outside looking in. He also recounts his own experience with masking. Autism is a rich source of originality and beauty for Byron D. Johnson and many others. Unfortunately, living in a neurotypical world can result in a great deal of misery and estrangement. Most Autistic people who wear masks struggle for years before realizing who they are. Additionally, they are more likely to be discriminated against because of their ethnicity, gender, sexual orientation, class, etc. Characteristics that add to their pain and make them invisible. Byron D. Johnson lays out the foundation for uncovering and provides activities that promote self-expression, such as:

- Celebrating unusual interests.

-Fostering relationships with people who are autistic.

- And rediscovering your values.

Chapter 1

What is autism, exactly?

ASD commonly referred to as autism spectrum disorder, is a type of developmental condition brought on by alterations in the brain. It is recognized that some people with autism have a difference, such as a genetic issue. Other factors aren't sure at this point. Researchers have hypothesized that there may be more than one factor contributing to the development of autism spectrum disorder, and these factors may interact with one another. We have much more to understand about these reasons and how they affect persons with autism spectrum disorder (ASD).

People with autism spectrum disorder (ASD), a neurodevelopmental condition, behave, speak, interact, and learn differently from most people. They often don't have any distinguishing features that set them apart from other folks. People with autism spectrum disorder may have various abilities (ASD). For instance, while some people with ASD are nonverbal, others may have highly developed communication skills. While some people with autism spectrum disorder (ASD) need a lot of help in their daily lives, others can live and work independently.

Typically, autism spectrum disorder (ASD) symptoms appear before age three. It may continue throughout a person's entire life, although some symptoms may become less severe as time passes. Within the first year of life, some children display symptoms of autism spectrum disorder (ASD). In certain circumstances, symptoms might not show up until 24 months of age or later. Until 18 and 24 months old, some kids with autism spectrum disorder (ASD) continue learning new things and hitting developmental milestones. At this time, students either stop learning new talents or stop using their prior skills.

When children with autism spectrum disorder mature into teenagers and young adults, they could struggle to make and keep friends, communicate with peers and adults, or comprehend what is expected of them in the classroom or at work. They may attract the attention of healthcare practitioners because they also suffer from disorders such as anxiety, depression, or attention-deficit/hyperactivity disorder, all of which are more prevalent in individuals with ASD than in individuals who do not have ASD.

Indicators and Indications

People with autism spectrum disorders frequently struggle with social communication, interaction, and limited or monotonous activities or hobbies. People with autism spectrum disorder (ASD) may also have distinct approaches to learning, movement, or paying attention. It is essential to remember that some persons who do not have ASD may also have some of these symptoms. For those with autism spectrum condition, these characteristics can make life incredibly challenging (ASD).Since autism is a neurological condition that lasts a person's entire life., People with autism interact with and experience the environment in a manner distinct from those who do not have autism.

The concept of neurodiversity enlightens us on the reality that variances in how the human brain functions occur naturally. Autism is an excellent example of neurodiversity, and as such, it ought to be regarded as a natural variation. It should be encouraged rather than a disorder that ought to be addressed.

Autism can be considered a spectrum, and each autistic person has distinct advantages and disadvantages. There are commonalities among autistic people, although each autistic person has their own unique experience of autism. The most significant dissimilarity aspects are related to communication and language differences.

Differences in terms of social interaction

• Behaviors, hobbies, and interests that are rigid

and repetitive.

• Differences in sensory perception.

What exactly is meant by the term "autistic masking"?

The act of concealing or denying aspects of a person's autistic identity or experience is called autistic masking. As an individual who supports autistic children in an educational context (or at home), you must be aware of why some children may hide their requirements.When it comes to autistic masking, research is just getting started, although it is estimated that 94 percent of autistic adults have done it at some point in their lives. When someone suppresses or hides aspects of their autism identity, this behavior is referred to as autistic masking. It is consciously or unconsciously and is commonly referred to as a "social survival strategy." It is employed to comply with the "norms" that are required of one, to cope with specific events or environments, or to prevent oneself from exhibiting discomfort.

In order to explain the concept of masking; a typical example is Superman's secret identity, Clark Kent. Superman is aware that he is unique and that, to 'fit in' with society, he must hide his unique qualities and create an unassuming and unremarkable role — he must be someone that no one will notice.It is possible that autistic masking is a reaction to the trauma and discrimination that autistic people face. The possibility that autistic persons require a social survival strategy indicates that society does not adequately supply their requirements.We learn to avoid being excluded, marginalized, invalidated and treated poorly. We must be "acceptable" and project a personality that gives others comfort so that we are not treated in such a manner. We can only avoid being excluded, marginalized, invalidated, and treated poorly.

Although more people are becoming aware of autism, there is still room for improvement in understanding and acceptance. According to a National Autistic Society study, 79% of autistic people reported feeling alienated due to a lack of knowledge of autism among the general public. The amount of effort required to mask something can be taxing. Maintaining a masking behavior for an extended period can harm mental health and well-being, although autistic persons may find temporary masking helpful in the present.

Chapter 2

The price that is paid to conceal autism

People with autism frequently mention that pretending to be someone else is tiring. The ability to conceal autism symptoms calls for a significant amount of: "effort," "concentration," "discomfort," and "self-control."

The effort that autistic people spend on disguising further depletes the resources available to manage their emotions and relationships with others. All of these things can make preexisting mental health problems much worse. Masking is linked to increased generalized and social anxiety and depression symptoms, and this association holds across gender lines. According to the findings of one study, people who admitted to using masking also had more excellent rates of suicide ideation. People with autism also describe experiencing great worry and tension after having their natural behaviors suppressed for an extended period. They then require time alone to discharge the behaviors they had been hiding.

When you mask your true self, there is a greater chance that your unique requirements may be disregarded or misinterpreted. It can result in a missed diagnosis or one received too late. It is also possible for people to perceive that they are not their true selves due to it. The more you hide who you are, the less likely people will understand and accept you for who you are.

Why does autism masquerade as something else? Individuals who are autistic have the potential to develop masking as a natural and adaptive response to the stresses that come with interacting in an environment that is not neurotypical. It is an attempt at connection, acceptance, and fitting in with the group.

In addition, it is a method for avoiding unfavorable responses and prejudice. If autistic individuals rely on their natural or intuitive social behaviors, they are much more likely to receive adverse reactions. Autism has always been viewed as a collection of challenges to be conquered. It is also considered a disorder that can be "cured." For instance, the primary focus of the therapy that autistic people receive is on modifying their actions to be perceived as capable and capable of performing tasks. This perspective on autism always results in stigma and exclusion for those who hold it.

People who do not have autism sometimes have a poor opinion of the characteristics linked with autism. When autistic individuals do not attempt to conceal their condition, they are more likely to face exclusion, bullying, or even physical assault.

People who have autism, on the other hand, often make an effort to conceal characteristics that are considered undesirable, even if doing so compromises their health. They are under the impression that to gain access to jobs and opportunities, they need to "fit in."

How prevalent is the practice of masking among people who have autism?

Only in more recent years has the phenomenon of masking been investigated. At this time, we only have a limited amount of data to show how widespread it is. However, in one research, seventy percent of autistic individuals said they try to blend in with their surroundings.It would indicate that autistic females can better conceal their condition than autistic males, often to survive in professional or educational contexts.

Both men and women admit to hiding aspects of themselves to socialize more easily or feel more accepted by their peers. To blend in with their peers, individuals who are neurodiverse in other ways, such as those with attention-deficit hyperactivity disorder (ADHD) or a learning handicap, may also resort to masking.

Examples of Autism's Disguising Behavior

The act of masking can take on a wide variety of forms. An individual may employ these methods consciously or unconsciously depending on the circumstances they find themselves. It is essential to remember that autistic masking is not the same as a non-autistic person utilizing short-term social techniques in stressful events, such as behaving more confidently than they feel in preparation for an effective presentation.

A person who engages in autistic masking may, at times over an extended period, deny significant aspects of their identity. For instance, they may pretend not to experience severe fear in response to particular sensory events.Mimicking other people's social behavior, such as their gestures or facial expressions, is one example of masking used, but the list is not exhaustive.Intentionally forcibly maintaining eye contact during conversations or pretending to do so. They are attempting to conceal or downplay the intensity of their interests.

Building a store of "stock phrases" for discussions and scripting or practicing dialogues, respectively. We are reducing or eliminating self-stimulatory behaviors (also known as "stimming").People with autism often engage in repetitive behaviors, such as whistling, leaping, clicking their fingers, etc., for various reasons, including to help themselves self-regulate and for fun.

Internalizing the unpleasantness of sensory input

Masking does not discriminate based on gender; however, it is hypothesized that one of the reasons that fewer females are currently being diagnosed with autism may be due to exceptionally high levels of masking in those who have a more internal presentation of autism – which those raised as girls make up a high proportion. In other words, masking may be one of the reasons why fewer females are being diagnosed.

Chapter 3

A Reassessment of Autism

Autism is typically presented as a handicap, and mainstream theories of autism use deficiency models to describe the condition. The iterative nature of research and the scientific method is sometimes glossed over when popular theories are presented as irrefutable evidence. Most conventional theories are mute regarding autistic talents and atypical abilities; in fact, what is written frequently paints a negative image of autism as an "epidemic." The use of hurtful phrases such as risk, disease, disorder, impairment, deficit, pedantic, and obsessive is daily. A recent genetic study that included identical and non-identical twins found that 56-95% of the observed features have a genetic basis; autism can be attributed to genetic differences that are referred to as polymorphisms. There is no such thing as a patent for perfect human genetics because there is a natural variation in the genetic makeup of individuals, families, and populations. Changes in a species' genetic makeup can occur continuously; when those changes are beneficial, they are carried forward to subsequent generations. The condition known as autism is an illustration of natural variation. Around 641,000 persons in Britain fall on the autism spectrum, corresponding to the current estimation that 1 in 100 people fall somewhere on the spectrum. Why do autistic variants of genes continue to be passed down if autism is, in fact, a disease or other harmful condition? Why don't you ask the security services in the United Kingdom? They presently hire ten percent of their workforce from our "neurodiverse" community, which includes persons on the autism spectrum. The pharmaceutical sector is the primary funder of the ongoing autism research that focuses on developing medical treatment options into medications, cures, and prenatal screening. This kind of program creates a lot of concerns, not the least of which is that autistic persons frequently fight for the right to be valued as equal but unique members of society, thereby challenging the concept of handicap. Due to it, there is apprehension when it is considered that the pharmaceutical business, which has a financial stake in maintaining a "disease model" of autism to make a profit in the future, would be involved with such research. Only one percent of people in the population would need treatment since their humanity would be reduced to symptoms. It seems like an easy pitch: first, convince everyone else that this group is a problem, and then convince the people you're trying to reach. People with autism are not tragedies in and of themselves. There is meaning and happiness in my life.

The idea that intellectual handicaps and autism are intimately related is widely held yet incorrectly believed. Despite this, many of the world's most influential intellectuals and innovators had autistic tendencies. "Autism and intellectual disability frequently co-occur in clinical settings, leading many academics to hypothesize that the same hereditary factors must cause the disorders. People with autism have a spectrum of intellectual abilities, ranging from average to superior intelligence. One plausible explanation for this disparity is that people with high levels of intellectual capacity are less likely to be diagnosed with autism. In addition, some diagnosticians deliberately avoid making a diagnosis in patients who appear to be managing their symptoms well. Whether or not they have received a diagnosis, a person with autism is aware that they are unique and have the right to be aware that they belong to a distinct minority group. The traditional representation of autism is inaccurate. 75% of persons who have autism can communicate verbally, and learning difficulty should not be confused with autism. Most people will know at least one autistic person, but that person may be unaware that they have the condition.

People with autism are human beings; they are genetically and neurologically diverse, but they are still people who think and feel. People with autism have strengths, struggles outside the norm, and divergent intuitive learning and communication styles. There is a tendency for society to be close-minded and excessively conformist.

One would have a hard time finding an autistic individual who has happy recollections of school because most autistic students are bullied by their peers. When they become adults, many people live in seclusion because their societies view them as "strange," "odd," and worthless. Because they have been socialized to speak and act in a manner that is foreign to them but conforms to what everyone else expects of them, many people who are highly educated and successful find the idea of "coming out" to be a scary proposition. Knowing that the world does not regard them for who they are is a draining and terrible experience for them. The conventional wisdom holds that autistic individuals may be more predisposed to mental health problems than the general community. One could guess that an abusive childhood, being an outsider in one's community, and hiding in the closet would be a hint at the reason. Autistic individuals are, after all, human. On the vast genetic tree that we all share, autism is an evolutionary offshoot. The European convention on human rights recognizes autistic people as a vulnerable minority group deserving of protection. Apathy is the enemy of progress, and while we sleep, big business may pre-natally diagnose, abort, treat, and "cure" an essential human group out of existence. Human rights appear to be of no concern when the person in issue has a label pinned to them indicating that they have a disability. We must unite to combat this injustice and establish autistic people as a distinct minority group. Please make an effort to include autistic people in society and recognize them for their genuine and significant contributions to the community. What is the use of studying history if we do not apply the things we find out?

Chapter 4

Creating a Life as an Autistic Person

Autism spectrum disorder (ASD) is a form of neurodivergence that affects males and male children to a far greater extent than it does females and female children.

Variances characterize autism in the way in which the brain is wired as well as how it functions. Although it is a disability, it does not imply deficiencies in persons considered neurotypical. Instead, it indicates that different levels of support and accommodations may be necessary for a person to flourish in their environment.

The process of getting a diagnosis can frequently

be very stressful. Understanding that autism is not a disease that requires treatment to be cured is essential. It indicates that individuals may need a diverse set of supports, modifications in their surroundings, and coping skills to live whole lives with minimal disturbances to their day-to-day functioning.

Autism denotes a neurodevelopmental difference. Some of these distinctions may be more obvious than others. In this case, adjusting a person's routines and environs may be necessary to provide them with the resources they require to function optimally.

This article examines the psychological, physiological, and social effects of living with autism spectrum disorder (ASD). Additionally, it offers advice to persons caring for someone with autism spectrum disorder (ASD).

Advice on Coping Emotionally While Living With Autism

According to research, autistic individuals are more likely to experience sensations of anxiety and tension, which can harm their emotional health, coping ability, and stress resistance. The expectations of society, which frequently urge that neurodiverse people must adhere to the requirements of neurotypical society, are the source of some of these pressures. People with autism struggle with difficulties even into adulthood, although the primary signs of autism appear throughout childhood. After a lifetime of living with the symptoms of an illness they didn't know they had, it can be challenging for an adult who is autistic to finally acquire a diagnosis after being misdiagnosed for so long. An explanation and a greater understanding of which supportive resources could be the most beneficial can be of assistance.

Gain an Understanding of the Emotional Obstacles

Autism is a form of neurodivergence, which implies that a person's brain functions in a manner that is not consistent with what is understood to be the neurotypical pattern. On the other hand, neurodivergent persons are frequently expected to think, act, and feel in ways typical of neurotypical people can contribute to emotional difficulties in day-to-day life. These emotional reactions may frequently be mistaken for other mental health illnesses, such as depression; additionally, the two conditions may sometimes coincide. Autism may also arise with other diseases, such as attention deficit hyperactivity disorder (ADHD), anxiety, sleep, or gastrointestinal difficulties.

Autistic persons have different ways of processing and conveying their emotions, making dealing with the feelings that come with an autism spectrum disorder diagnosis even more challenging.

Discover Methods to Control Your Anxiety

A significant portion of autistic people struggles with anxiety. This kind of anxiety may result from difficulties associated with day-to-day living. Still, it may also result from apprehensions regarding interactions with other people, challenges in adapting to novel settings or pursuits, or feelings of alienation from those with whom the individual is familiar. If you have anxiety symptoms, it is vital to assess if these sensations result from a transient condition (such as a recent change in your life) or whether they could result from an anxiety disorder. Feeling that other people don't get you might also contribute to anxiety. Challenges in communication,

particularly for people who are non-verbal, can also contribute to feelings of anxiousness in some people. Utilize relaxation techniques such as a weighted blanket, creating art, going for a walk, using a fidget toy, engaging in breathing exercises, or utilizing a fidget spinner.

Keeping Your Health in Check While Dealing With Autism

When autistic persons go to the doctor, their condition will likely continue to be a central topic of discussion during the entire visit. However, it is essential to maintain other regular medical examinations, such as annual physicals and monthly dentist appointments.

Keeping a schedule and engaging in self-care are two helpful strategies we can utilize. Finding a plan to maintain a consistent pattern can be beneficial for persons with autism, as the disorder makes it more challenging for them to cope with changes in their routine.

Develop a daily schedule that includes regular sleeping hours, standard meal times, self-care activities, and home responsibilities. Engaging in self-care activities such as regular exercise, taking breaks to rest, and practicing stress management is crucial.

The Benefits of Living an Active Lifestyle

More than one therapy option is available for persons with autism spectrum disorder (ASD). A relatively small number of these regimens involve some exercise routine. Some persons who have autism spectrum disorder (ASD) may discover that their motor abilities, such as walking or coordination, are impaired.

According to some research, autistic children can benefit from better communication and behavior if they engage in activities that require them to move around. If you have autism, one of the essential things you can do for your health is to find activities you enjoy doing to keep active. Eating a healthy, balanced diet, being active consistently, and getting adequate sleep are all essential components of any effective treatment plan, including medication and psychotherapy.

Keeping a Healthy and Well-Balanced Diet

Because of difficulties with food textures, odors, and other sensory experiences, some autistic people have problems following a balanced diet. For instance, individuals can have trouble eating some foods because they are hypersensitive to the colors, tastes, or textures of those items.

It is necessary to find ways to work around these dietary preferences to locate foods that a person likes that are also nutritious. It may take some work, but it is essential to find ways to do so. It may also require patience and some trial and error, so you should be prepared to test a variety of meals, most of which you will most likely reject before you find some foods suitable for your diet. You can create a meal plan based on the meals you liked and disliked in a food journal that you keep for yourself or someone important to you.

Sleep Challenges

In addition, some autistic individuals have trouble falling or staying asleep.

It can be brought on by various factors, from an inability to settle down to being overstimulated. If you have autism and find it challenging to get enough sleep, sticking to a tight bedtime schedule will benefit you. It is especially true if you have trouble falling asleep. Maintain a sleep log in which you note the days you have difficulty falling asleep and what you suspect may be the cause.

Chapter 5

Developing Relationships with Autistic People

In the previous few years, numerous individuals have pondered how they may make their surroundings more accessible to people with autism. Architects have published articles on autism-friendly architecture design, and families have remodeled their homes to provide stimulating sensory experiences for autistic family members.

Listening to persons who have a condition that falls somewhere on the autism spectrum makes it abundantly evident that their experiences of the

world might be entirely dissimilar to those of others. It has the potential to be both a handicap and an advantage. To make the environment more accessible to people with autism, we need to work to mitigate the unfavorable consequences of sensory impairments while amplifying the favorable effects. As a result of the fact that every person on the autism spectrum will have a unique sensory experience of the world, the following ideas are intended to be taken as broad guidelines, and special consideration should be given to each individual's preferences wherever it is feasible to do so. There are some questions that we have to ask ourselves. There are some questions that we should be asking ourselves before we start the process of remodeling a room or designing a building to assist in determining how we will go about making adjustments that will be beneficial for people who

have autism. We can find these questions here. To answer many of these issues, you must analyze the existing environment, consider the seven sense markers, and pay close attention to the individuals using the domain. When asking questions about the senses, it is essential to keep in mind that people with autism can either be hypersensitive (get an excessive amount of sensory information) or hyposensitive (receive insufficient amounts of sensory information) (receive too little sensory information). They may also be hypersensitive or hyposensitive, requiring a smaller stimulus response but a more extensive reply at other times. When we are attempting to make the surrounding world more accessible for people with autism, some questions that we need to ask ourselves include the following:

1. Visual sense (Sight)

2. The sense of hearing (Hearing)

3. The ability to feel both pressure and touch

4. Sensation of smell or odor (Smell)

5. Taste sense

6.Vestibular sense (Balance)

7. Proprioceptive sense (Space)

8. Who is going to make use of the space?

9. For what purposes will the area be utilized?

Questions about the reception of visual information

How bright is each room, both naturally and with artificial lighting?

What color is the wall paint?

How many objects do you think there are in this room that requires you to have visual awareness or recognition?

Are there any patterns on the carpets, curtains, or

other furnishings?

The lighting significantly impacts the sensory experiences of many autistic people in their environments. Because some people can see the flashing of fluorescent lights at a rate of sixty flashes per second, we now know that these lights can be pretty distracting, even incapacitating, for some individuals (60Hz). Some fluorescent light bulbs have a flicker rate of 120 Hz.

Natural illumination is another factor, particularly when it comes to establishing healthy sleeping patterns. Melatonin is a hormone that has a role in the regulation of sleep and waking cycles. It is one of the reasons why. In most cases, melatonin levels rise at night and fall during the daytime hours. If a person with autism has trouble sleeping, one of the numerous tactics we can try is to ensure that there is complete darkness during the periods when they

are supposed to be sleeping. The importance of paying attention to color cannot be overstated. We respond differently to various colors for a variety of reasons. As an illustration, the color red has the longest wavelength, and as a consequence, it has the potential to excite us and quicken our heart rate. Yellow is another color with a long wavelength that can stimulate. The mind can be put at ease and focus improved by wearing light blues. The color green can be calming. Think about the room you are decorating; are you attempting to create a stimulating or calming environment? Consideration must also be given to the degree to which the rooms are congested or uncluttered.

Many people with autism are hyper-aware of their surroundings and can easily get overwhelmed when confronted with excessive visual information to assimilate. Some people require more stimulus

from the visual arts. Fabrics with patterns might be very upsetting to some people who suffer from conditions that fall under the autism spectrum. Prints can be disorienting and overwhelming and cause visual distortion if they are not appropriately handled.

Questions about the reception of sounds

Are there consistent sounds from the outside, such as passing cars, children playing, or construction?

Are there any reoccurring noises within the building, such as clocks ticking, the humming of refrigerators, or music?

Is it possible to lessen the amount of noise that

comes from the outside and makes its way inside? Do you know how to lower the loudness of the sounds that each person hears, such as using earplugs?

Many individuals with autism have reported to us that they can hear sounds several decibels louder than those that others can listen to. They can hear sounds far further away, and the volume of the sounds might overwhelm them. They can have loud rock music playing in the background while still being able to hear a conversation taking place in the room next door.

Concerning issues of contact and exertion-related issues

Is there a location offering various surfaces that can be touched and stroked?

I was wondering if there are things that can produce varied sensations on the skin, such as sand or water.

Is there anything that can offer pressure if it's required, like a wooden massager or something?

Some persons who have autism avoid physical contact unless they can exert some control over it. Others require additional pressure to feel peaceful and comfortable, and they can benefit from using objects such as weighted blankets, provided they are appropriately utilized. If a person is very hyposensitive, they may require further stimulus to feel anything (filter out too much sensory information instead of too little).

Concerning the scent sense, the questions that follow (Olfactory)

Is it possible to detect any odors outside the room or building thanks to the building's construction, windows, or doors?

Are odors coming from the house, such as those of cleaning agents, perfumed goods, or foods, that have the potential to be upsetting?

Smells can be pretty overwhelming for some people with autism, and as a result, they experience intense nausea. Some people will continue to smell the product for a considerable time, even when it is removed from the room or cabinet.

Questions on the sense of taste

When designing an environment in which the sense of taste will be utilized, such as a dining room, it is crucial to remember that sometimes we can assume a distaste for a flavor when it could be caused by something else. It is something that should be kept in mind when designing the environment. An unpleasant sensation caused by the meal's texture or the food's appearance could be the source of an unpleasant taste. Questions to ponder include, "Have we established a setting in which individuals have access to easily discernible choices?"

Are there pictures to accompany the words describing the many cuisine options?

Questions about the sense of balance (vestibular) and the surrounding environment (proprioceptive)

I'm wondering whether there are any prospects for swinging.

Is there a chance to practice maintaining your balance on beams or boards?

Are there any opportunities to climb or bounce?

Is there any way for a person to sit with their back against a wall if they want to?

Is there any seating available from which a person could see the room?

·Are there rapid exit routes?

Some autistic persons have trouble having a sense of themselves in connection to the physical

environment around them, and this can be pretty challenging for them. By rocking, swinging, or balancing, they might better understand who they are. If they need something directly behind them or in front of them to obtain a sense of who they are, having too much space in front of them or behind them can induce anxiety. Additionally, some people with autism experience stress if they cannot see what is occurring or where sounds are coming from, which they find very disorienting. It can cause them to feel helpless or trapped.

Many individuals who have autism require space around them and get anxious when confronted with crowds or clutter. The maze of passageways can make them feel trapped, so they must be reassured that there is a speedy way out.

Who is going to make use of the space?

Although this may appear to be a silly question, it is essential to consider the response carefully. Likely, the atmosphere needs to be adjusted for adults but not kids. You might also need to examine whether the same area will be used by other people who could have different sensory needs or by a group of people whose sensory requirements are substantially different from one another. Is there another location a person can go to get away from all of the stimulation if there is a chance that they would have sensory overload?

What sorts of activities are planned for the room? Some rooms, like auditoriums in schools or open-concept workplaces, are designed to accommodate many people simultaneously. The remaining areas are designated for individual use or use by small groups. However, other areas, such as corridors or

lifts, are designed specifically for transition. Since moving from one place or activity to another is not always straightforward, autistic people may have trouble navigating transitional areas. As a result, it is necessary to give some thought to the question of how transition spaces can be made less challenging to navigate. You might want to consider things like, "Is it possible for there to be a natural flow from one space to another without using corridors?" Is there a less claustrophobic way to walk up or down a building than the lifts provided?

If there are spaces available, but big groups of people are using them, are smaller locations that can be used as a retreat if necessary?

Are there possibilities to readily get to a more open environment, even if the spaces are tiny and intimate?

Can you make a map showing where people with autism experience the most anxiety? Are there any other possible ways to get there?

Chapter 6

Developing a Society Comprised of Neurodiversity

Everyone is considered part of the neurodiversity community, regardless of whether they are neurotypical (defined as having neurological functioning that is considered to be "average") or neurodivergent (who fall outside this). Autism, attention deficit hyperactivity disorder (ADHD), dyslexia, and dyspraxia or attention deficit hyperactivity disorder (DCD) are all examples of neurodivergence.

Adjusting to the surrounding environment

1. The environment that stimulates the senses Is there a location for everyone to work where they may relax and be productive? Is it possible to concentrate despite distracting sights, scents, and sounds? Is there enough light in the room? What about unpleasant sensations to the sense of touch? Have you thought about the configuration of the room? Can we implement any measures to make the working environment more comfortable? Whoever needs them should have free access to earplugs, computer screen filters, and room dividers, if possible. Have specific sensitivities to the surroundings, such as solid perfume, been considered, and do other people understand why this is important?

2. The appropriate circumstances Have the tasks

been given the necessary time? We can increase our success by allowing time to reflect on lessons and address those activities appropriately. Are time scales realistic? Have there been conversations about them? Are there definite protocols to follow if tasks are completed ahead of schedule or need more time? Is the number of times you're asked to do things quickly kept to a minimum, and do you have the option to decline being required to answer quickly?

3. The environment that is made clear. Is there a clear indication of all that needs to be done in a task? Are any functions that rely on an implicit understanding that draws upon societal norms or the customary expectations of a particular situation? Is it obvious which responsibilities ought to take precedence over others? A check to ensure that

everything has been made clear may help avoid uncertainty later. Avoid coming across as condescending. Is there a predetermined process for asking questions if they become necessary, such as a designated person (a mentor) to approach at the beginning?

4. The environment that we can anticipate In what ways is the environment unpredictable? The maximum level of predictability—is it even possible? A predictable atmosphere can assist reduce anxiety and make concentrating on the task easier. Uncertainty is known to be an anxiety-inducing factor. Is it possible to schedule recurring meetings? Is it feasible that we will need to postpone or cancel some of our meetings in the future? Are the policies for handling the cancellation of anticipated events (such discussions)

and the justifications for any changes understood? Is it possible to receive resources and materials in advance?

5. The surrounding social context Does the setting provide opportunities for social interaction, and how willing or hesitant is everyone to take part in those opportunities? Exist mandatory gatherings of friends and family? Can the group's activities be altered so that everyone can take part in them? For instance, the invitation might be worded more clearly and directed toward a specific event with a set time limit. Does everybody in the setting understand that not wanting to interact with others socially does not necessarily mean that one does not like them or is nasty to them? Would it be beneficial for people to have a traffic-light system (for example, green, yellow, or red post-it notes) to

signify their readiness to connect with others and their present stress level? You can determine the degree to which the environment is Sensory, Timely, Explicit, and Predictable by considering the "Reasonable Adjustment STEPS" model.

Providing Assistance to Individuals

6. Disclosing diagnosis Are individuals willing to reveal any diagnosis they may have to their coworkers, and if yes, how would they wish this situation to be handled? Would the individuals who work with the individual benefit from training or the chance to ask questions? In that case, is it possible to involve a reliable third party who is impartial to facilitate an honest and cordial conversation? If the person gives the information to their coworkers, are they willing for their coworkers to share the information with additional

individuals, or is this information considered confidential? As an illustration, when the topic of autism comes up in discussion, it is crucial to find out the language the individual prefers to communicate in. (for example, a person with autism, an Aspie, autistic, or a person with autism)

7. Problems with Planning, Flexibility, Sustained Attention, or Inertia During Project Management. Does Anyone Else Experience These Issues? What factors contribute to the worsening of these challenges, and how may they be mitigated? Exist any online resources (such programs for time management or shared calendars, for example) that could be able to lend the project some more structure? Which of the staff members would prefer a non-linear planning system (such as mind maps or sketch notes) as opposed to a linear planning

system (such as a Gantt chart or a "to-do" list), and is it possible to accommodate this preference? Which individuals would prefer to be wholly immersed in a particular subject or activity, as opposed to having a selection of multiple assignments with varying intermediate deadlines, and can this choice be included in the work plan for the project?

8. Different modes of communication Is there anyone who favors more literal and specific language? Can they remind their line manager, supervisor, and coworkers to use this if that's the case? Which mode of communication, face-to-face or written, is more prevalent among people? Is it simpler to talk on Skype than it is on the phone? Should coworkers be reminded to explain why they are making a specific comment or advice and

provide the statement itself? Is there an environment where they feel comfortable approaching their line manager, supervisor, or colleagues for assistance when they have a problem?

9. Health and wellness, as well as a healthy work-life balance. How well do folks appear to be sleeping and eating? Are the times of the meetings going to be convenient for their schedules? Can they work from home, or do their break times and working hours vary? Is everyone familiar with the pertinent services, such as those for people with disabilities or human resources? Is a primary care physician on file for them? Do they need to take a leave of absence due to their impairment to receive treatment or therapeutic support? Do they require assistance or recommendations from third-party services such as Access to Work or the Disabled

Students Allowance?

10. Identifying and fixing problems Do you have one-on-one meetings with each person to talk about what is going well and what may be improved? Is there a way that they can adapt the coping mechanisms that they use in other contexts so that they can utilize them here? The responsibilities that fall within the employment description or the course could be modified. Or, would it be possible to divide the job among the employees so that everyone could make the most of their skills? Collaborate to find new answers to problems that haven't been handled, and be prepared to deal with further issues if they appear.

Conclusion

For autistic persons to stop having to hide their needs, differences, and unique talents, it is time for increased societal acceptance and tolerance of difference. Autistic and neurotypical individuals can benefit from nonconformity and learn to live genuinely by embracing neurodiversity.